KETO COPYCAT RECIPES

Learn how to cook Step-by-Step all the tasty keto recipes from the world's most famous restaurants. The definitive cookbook to prepare comfortably at home best stars chef's dishes.

Lillie Logan

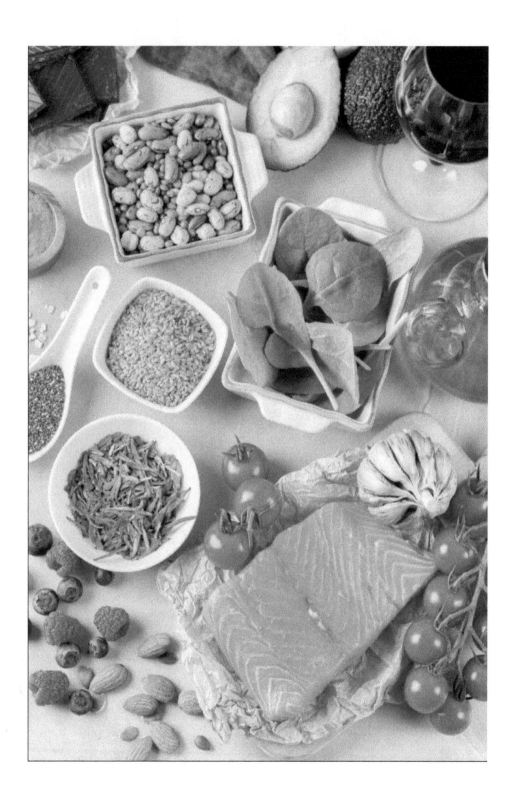

TABLE OF CONTENTS

Chapter 1

Keto copycat
Breakfast, Appetizers, Salads

Mcgriddle Sandwiches

PREPARATION: 15 MIN   **COOKING: 15 MIN**   **SERVING: 6**

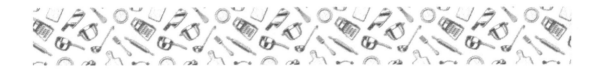

Ingredients:

Buns

1/2 cup sugar free pancake syrup

3 large eggs

3 oz. cream cheese

1 cup Almond Flour

2 tsp Baking Powder

1 1/2 tsp vanilla extract

1 tsp maple extract

1/2 tsp liquid stevia

Filling

6 Large Eggs

Salt and Pepper to taste

6 slices cheese

6 slices bacon or sausage cooked

Directions:

Over medium-high heat, heat the syrup to a boil in a saucepan, stir constantly. Boil until syrup becomes thick and reduced by half. Pour the syrup on a parchment lined pan and place in freezer for at least 1 hour.

Preheat oven to 350 °F and line a cookie sheet with foil and place 12 mason jar rings onto the pan (or grease a 12-cavity whoopie pie pan). Spray the inside of the rings with non-stick spray.

Place the remaining ingredients for the buns into a blender and pulse until smooth. Pour evenly into the rings (approximately 2-3 tbsp. per lid)

Remove the syrup from the freezer and gently peel the parchment or foil away from the syrup. cut it into small pieces and evenly distribute the pieces into the batter.

Bake for 12-15 minutes, or until set. Allow to cool slightly before removing from the rings or the whoopie pie pan.

For the Eggs: You can make them fried or scrambled based upon your preference. I like to bake the eggs to make them like a real fast food sandwich. Just beat the eggs with salt and pepper, then pour into a greased 7×11 or 9×13 baking dish and bake in the preheated oven for about 15 minutes or until the eggs are set. Allow them to cool, then slice into 6 even pieces.

Assemble the sandwiches by topping one pancake bun with one slice of bacon or sausage, one egg and one slice of cheese, then top with a second bun.

Nutrition:

Calories: 374kcal

Carbohydrates: 6g

Protein: 19g

Fat: 29g

Saturated Fat: 9g

Cholesterol: 287mg

Sodium: 384mg

Potassium: 349mg

Fiber: 4g

Sugar: 1g

Vitamin A: 825IU

Calcium: 366mg

Iron: 2.3mg

Waffles

PREPARATION: 10 MIN

COOKING: 20 MIN

SERVING: 5

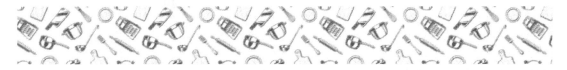

Ingredients:

5 eggs – medium separated

4 tbsp. coconut flour

4 tbsp. granulated sweetener of choice or more, to taste

1 tsp baking powder

2 tsp vanilla

3 tbsp. full fat milk or cream

125 g butter melted

Directions:

1st bowl

Whisk the egg whites until it becomes firm and form stiff peaks.

2nd bowl

Mix coconut flour, egg yolks, baking powder, and sweetener.

Slowly add the melted butter, continuously mix to ensure a smooth consistency.

Add the milk and vanilla, then mix well.

Fold spoons of the whisked egg whites gently to the yolk mixture. Try to keep the air and fluffiness as much as possible.

Put enough waffle mixture into the warm waffle maker. Cook until golden.

Repeat cooking in the waffle maker until all mixture is used.

Nutrition:

1. Calories 280
2. Calories from Fat 234
3. Fat 26g
4. Total Carbohydrates 4.5g
5. Fiber 2g
6. Sugar 1.4g
7. Protein 7g
8. NET carbs 2.5g

Chicken Bites With Sweet Mustard Dipping Sauce (Chick-Fil-A)

PREPARATION: 1 hour 20 MIN

COOKING: 20 MIN

SERVING: 8

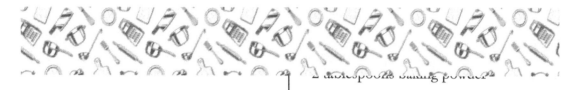

Ingredients:

For mustard sauce:

1 cup mayonnaise

4 teaspoons apple cider vinegar

½ teaspoon turmeric powder

20 – 30 drops liquid stevia

4 teaspoons Dijon mustard

1 teaspoon garlic powder

½ teaspoon onion powder

For chicken:

2 pounds hand-trimmed chicken breast, cut into 1-inch pieces

1 teaspoon coarse kosher salt

2 tablespoons baking powder

1 – 2 teaspoons salt or to taste

1 teaspoon paprika

Oil to fry, as required

2 – 4 tablespoons pickle juice

1 cup unflavored whey protein isolate

2 tablespoons erythritol

1 teaspoon garlic powder

1 teaspoon pepper

Directions:

To make mustard sauce: add all the ingredients for the mustard sauce into an airtight container and stir until well incorporated.

Cover the lid and refrigerate until use. It can last for 15 days.

11

To make chicken: add pickle juice and kosher salt into a large Ziploc bag. Seal the bag. Shake until well combined.

Add chicken and seal the bag. Shake the bag well. Chill for at least an hour. Turn the bag around for a couple of times during this time.

Take out the bag from the refrigerator 30 minutes before frying.

Place a deep fryer pan over medium flame. Pour enough oil in the pan and let the oil heat to 350° F.

Meanwhile, add whey protein powder, erythritol, garlic powder, pepper, baking powder, salt and paprika into a shallow bowl and stir well.

Dredge chicken pieces in the mixture, one at a time and place on a lined baking sheet.

Carefully add a few of the chicken bites in the hot oil. Turn the bites so that they are golden brown on all sides.

When golden brown, put onto a plate that is lined with paper towels.

Fry the remaining bites similarly.

Serve chicken bites with mustard sauce.

Tip: Serve chicken bites with Pink drink.

Nutrition:

For 1 tablespoon mustard dipping sauce:

Calories 92,

Fat 10 g,

Total Carbohydrate 0 g,

Net Carbohydrate 0 g,

Fiber 0 g,

Protein 10 g

4 ounces chicken bites:

Calories 284,

Fat 17 g,

Total Carbohydrate 3 g,

Net Carbohydrate 2 g,

Fiber 0 g,

Protein 34 g

Chicken Strips (Kfc)

 PREPARATION: 8 MIN   **COOKING: 5 – 6 MIN**   **SERVING: 6**

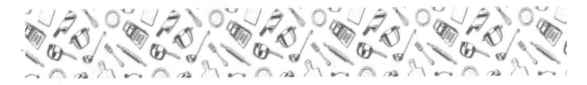

Ingredients:

2 chicken thighs, boneless, cut each into 3 pieces

1 ½ teaspoon KFC seasoning or to taste

Oil to fry, as required

¾ cup almond flour

1 egg, beaten

Directions:

Place a deep fryer pan over medium flame. Pour enough oil in the pan and let the oil heat to 350° F.

Meanwhile, add almond flour and KFC seasoning to a shallow bowl and stir well.

Dredge chicken pieces in the almond flour mixture, one at a time.

Next dip the chicken pieces in egg, shaking off the extra egg, dredge once again in almond flour mixture and place on a lined baking sheet.

Carefully add 2 – 3 of the chicken pieces in the hot oil. Cook until golden brown.

Remove chicken strips and place on a plate.

Fry the remaining chicken pieces similarly.

Tip: Serving the chicken strips with a Shamrock Shake will make it a complete meal.

Nutrition:

1. Calories 218,
2. Fat 17 g,
3. Total Carbohydrate 8 g,
4. Net Carbohydrate 4 g,
5. Fiber 4 g,
6. Protein 8 g

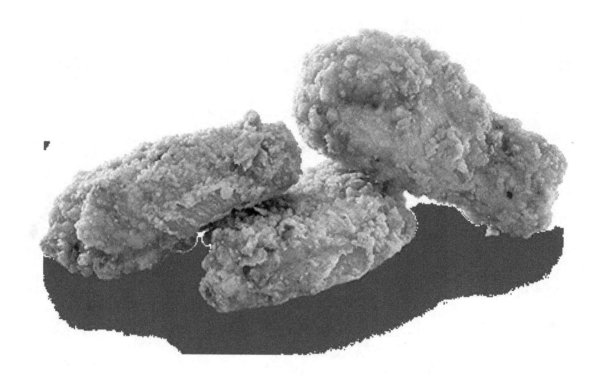

Potato Salad

PREPARATION: 5 MIN   **COOKING: 10 MIN**   **SERVING: 4**

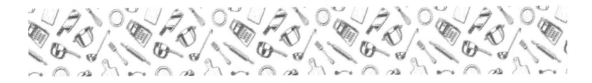

Ingredients:

6 cup cooked, cubed potatoes

¾ cup hooters wing sauce (Medium or Hot)

8 hard-boiled eggs, chopped

½ green pepper, diced

1 teaspoon black pepper

½ red pepper, diced

2 fresh scallions, minced

¾ cup mayonnaise

1 teaspoon seasoned salt

Directions:

Combine the entire ingredients together in a large bowl; mix well until nicely coated.

Serve immediately & enjoy.

Nutrition:

Calories: 628 kcal

Protein: 25.79 g

Fat: 33.97 g

Carbohydrates: 55.55 g

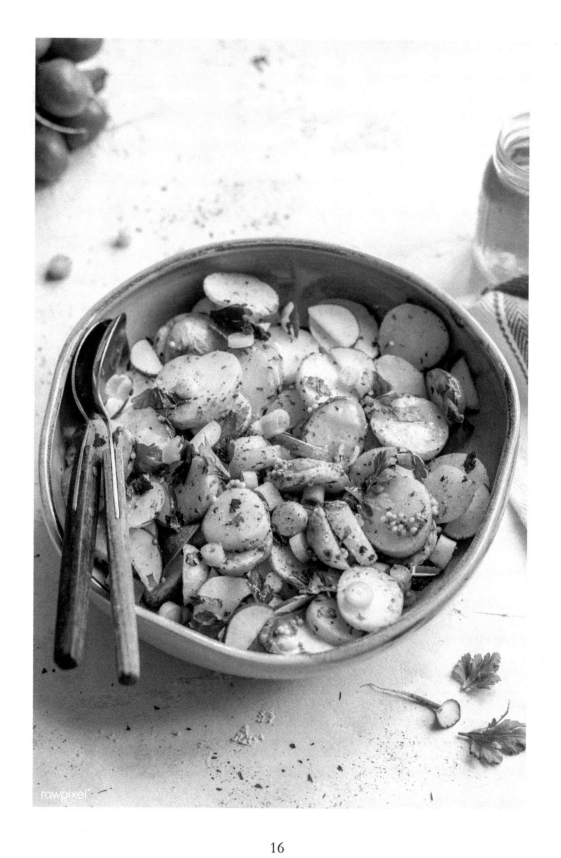

Chicken Garden Salad

PREPARATION: 35 MIN   **COOKING: 30 MIN**   **SERVING: 6**

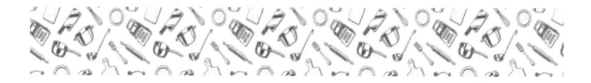

Ingredients:

1 pound asparagus spears, fresh

2 teaspoons garlic, finely chopped

1 pint (2 cups) grape tomatoes, cut in half

1 ½ teaspoons rosemary leaves, dried

1 teaspoon seasoned salt

6 boneless skinless chicken breasts (4 to 5 ounces each)

1 cup thinly sliced red onion

2 tablespoons canola or olive oil

1 bag (5 ounces) ready-to-eat spring mix salad greens

½ cup refrigerated honey Dijon dressing, reduced-fat

Directions:

Snap or cut off the tough ends from asparagus spears; place the spears in a shallow glass dish. Drizzle with 1 teaspoon of oil; turning several times until nicely coated. Cover & refrigerate until ready to grill.

Combine the leftover oil with garlic, rosemary & seasoned salt in a small bowl. On both sides of each chicken breast, rub it with the prepared oil mixture; place in a separate shallow dish. Cover & refrigerate for 30 minutes.

Heat a charcoal grill over moderate heat. Place the chicken on grill. Cover the grill & cook the chicken 15 to 20 minutes, turning a couple of times & adding asparagus after 7 minutes, until juice of chicken is clear when center of thickest part is cut. For 6 to 8 minutes, cook the asparagus until crisp-tender, turning frequently.

Cut asparagus into 1" pieces. Toss the asparagus with salad greens, onion and tomatoes in a large bowl. Put dressing on top of the salad; toss to coat. Cut chicken into strips; serve on top of the salad.

Nutrition:

Calories: 142 kcal

Protein: 2.23 g

Fat: 7.38 g

Carbohydrates: 19.31 g

Chapter 2
Keto Copycat Lunch

Longhorn's Parmesan Crusted Chicken

PREPARATION: 10 MIN   **COOKING: 30 MIN**   **SERVING: 4**

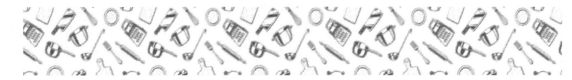

Ingredients:

4 chicken breasts, skinless

2 teaspoons salt

2 teaspoons ground black pepper

2 tablespoons avocado oil

For the Marinade:

1 tablespoon minced garlic

½ teaspoon ground black pepper

1 teaspoon lemon juice

3 tablespoon Worcestershire sauce

1 teaspoon white vinegar

½ cup avocado oil

½ cup ranch dressing

For the Parmesan Crust:

1 cup panko breadcrumbs

6 ounces parmesan cheese, chopped

5 tablespoons melted butter, unsalted

6 ounces provolone cheese, chopped

2 teaspoons garlic powder

6 tablespoons ranch salad dressing, low-carb

Directions:

Prepare the marinade and for this, take a small bowl, place all of its ingredients in it and then whisk until well combined.

Pound each chicken until ¾-inch thick, then season with salt and black pepper and transfer chicken pieces to a large plastic bag.

Pour in the prepared marinade, seal the bag, turn it upside to coat chicken with it. For at least 30 minutes, let it stay in the refrigerator.

Then take a large skillet pan, place it over medium-high heat, add oil and when hot, place marinated chicken breast in it and then cook for 5 minutes per side until chicken is no longer pink and nicely seared on all sides.

Transfer chicken to a plate and repeat with the remaining chicken pieces.

Meanwhile, switch on the oven, set it to 450 degrees F, and let it preheat.

When the chicken has cooked, prepare the parmesan crust and for this, take a small heatproof bowl, place both cheeses in it, pour in ranch dressing and milk, stir until mixed, and then microwave for 30 seconds.

Then stir the cheese mixture again until smooth and continue microwaving for another 15 seconds.

Stir the cheese mixture again, spread evenly on top of each chicken breast, arrange them in a baking sheet and then bake for 5 minutes until cheese has melted.

Meanwhile, take a small bowl, place breadcrumbs in it, stir in garlic powder and butter in it.

After 5 minutes of baking, spread the breadcrumbs mixture on top of the chicken and then continue baking for 2 minutes until the panko mixture turns light brown.

Serve chicken straight away with cauliflower mashed potatoes.

Nutritional Info:

Cal 557

Fats 42 g

Protein 31 g

Net Carb 10 g

Fiber 2 g

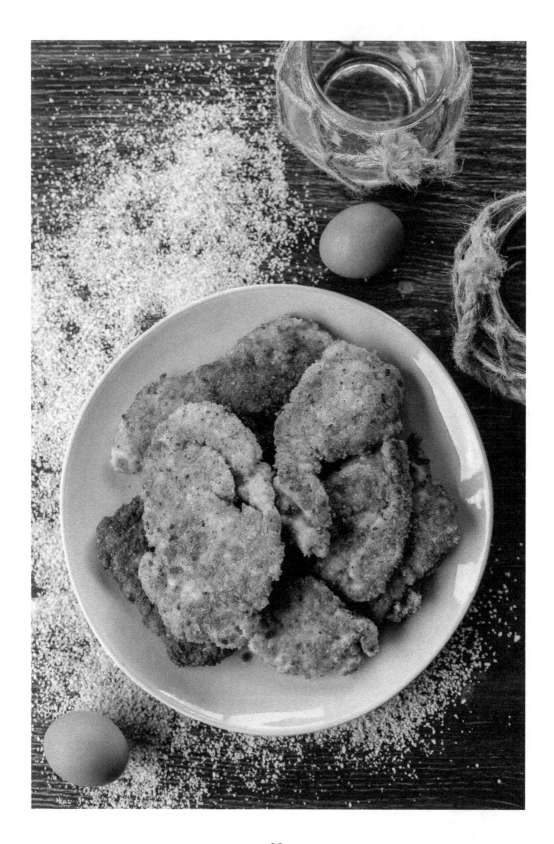

Panda Express Kung Pao Chicken

PREPARATION: 10 MIN

COOKING: 30 MIN

SERVING: 10

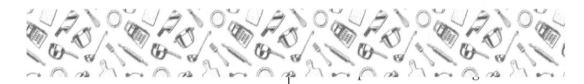

Ingredients:

35 ounces chicken thighs, skinless, ½-inch cubed

14 ounces zucchini, destemmed, ½-inch diced

14 ounces red bell pepper, cored, 1-inch cubed

1 green onion, sliced

15 pieces of dried Chinese red peppers

1 ½ teaspoons minced garlic

1 teaspoon minced ginger

3 ounces roasted peanuts

¼ teaspoon ground black pepper

¼ teaspoon xanthan gum

1 tablespoon chili garlic sauce

¾ tablespoon sesame oil

For the Marinade:

3 tablespoons coconut aminos

1 tablespoon coconut oil

For the Sauce:

3 tablespoons monk fruit sweetener

3 tablespoons coconut aminos

Directions:

Marinade the chicken and for this, take a large bowl, place the chicken pieces in it, and then add all the ingredients for the marinade in it.

Stir until chicken is well coated and then marinate for a minimum of 30 minutes in the refrigerator.

Then take a large skillet pan, add 1 tablespoon of coconut oil in it and when it melted, add marinated chicken and cook for 10 minutes or more until it starts to release its water.

After 10 minutes, push the chicken to the sides of the pan to create a well in its middle, slowly stir in xanthan gum into the water released by chicken and cook for 2 to 4 minutes until it starts to thicken.

Then stir chicken into the thicken liquid and continue cooking for 10 minutes or more until chicken has thoroughly cooked, set aside until required.

Return pan over medium-high heat, add 1 tablespoon oil, and when it melts, add bell pepper and zucchini cubes and then cook for 5 to 8 minutes until lightly browned.

Transfer vegetables to a separate plate, then add remaining coconut oil into the pan, add Chinese red peppers, ginger, garlic, vinegar, and chili garlic sauce.

Stir until mixed, cook for 3 minutes, add ingredients for the sauce along with peanuts, green onion, black pepper, and sesame oil and continue cooking for 3 minutes, stirring frequently.

Return chicken and vegetables into the pan, toss until well mixed and then continue cooking for 3 to 5 minutes until hot.

Serve straight away.

Nutritional Info:

Cal 295

Fats 16.4 g

Protein 31.7 g

Net Carb 3.2 g

Fiber 2 g

Chapter 3
Keto Copycat Dinner

Long John Silver's Batter-Dipped Fish

PREPARATION: 5 MIN

COOKING: 10 MIN

SERVING: 1/6

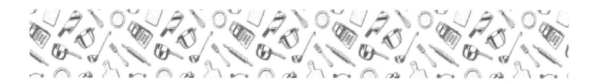

Ingredients:

4 cups vegetable oil (for frying)

2 pounds cod (cut into three-inch pieces)

16 ounces club soda

¼ cup ground flaxseed

2 cups almond flour

½ teaspoon paprika

½ teaspoon onion salt

½ teaspoon baking soda

½ teaspoon baking powder

1 teaspoon Himalayan sea salt

¼ teaspoon black pepper

Directions:

First, take a deep frying pan and fill it with the 4 cups of oil. Turn the heat to medium to preheat the oil.

As the oil heats, combine the almond flour and ground flaxseed with the paprika, onion salt, baking soda, baking powder, sea salt, and black pepper into a medium-sized mixing bowl. Whisk everything together so it is well incorporated, then add the club soda. Whisk again until the batter has a foamy consistency.

Take your cod pieces and dip them into your batter. Ensure that each piece is coated completely then carefully place them into the preheated oil. Do not overcrowd your pan or your fish will not cook evenly. If needed, fry in two batches. Allow the fish to fry for 5 minutes. The fish should have a nice golden color and will begin to float on the oil when done.

Remove the fish from the oil using a slotted spoon and transfer them to a plate lined with paper towels to catch the excess oil.

Serve with your favorite side!

Nutrition:

Calories 559

Carbs 2g

Fat 43g

Protein 37g

Olive Garden's Steak Gorgonzola Alfredo

PREPARATION: 20 MIN,   **COOKING: 25 MIN**   **SERVING: ¼**

20 MIN chill time

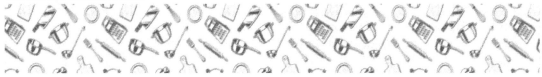

Ingredients:

1 pound of steak medallions

1 tablespoon balsamic vinegar

½ teaspoon Himalayan sea salt

½ teaspoon black pepper

5 zucchinis

4 ounces gorgonzola crumbles

¼ cup sun-dried tomatoes

For the Sauce

2 cups heavy cream

1 stick of unsalted butter

1 cup parmesan cheese

2 cups spinach

¼ teaspoon nutmeg

¼ teaspoon Himalayan sea salt

¼ teaspoon black pepper

Directions:

Begin by marinating your steaks. First, sprinkle them with the Himalayan sea salt and black pepper, then place them in a sealable bag. Add the balsamic vinegar to the bag and seal. Place the steaks in your refrigerator for at least 30 minutes before cooking

As the steaks marinate, place a large pot of water on your stovetop and turn the heat to medium high. Then take a spiralizer and create your "fettuccine noodles" using the zucchini. You can also use a vegetable peeler to peel thicker zoodles if you do not have a spiralizer. When done, add them to your boiling pot of water for 3 minutes. Then, drain the water and transfer your zucchini noodles to a plate lined with a paper towel, so the excess water can drain off.

Next, take a large skillet and place it on your stove. Turn the heat to medium and allow it to heat up. Remove your steak medallions and place them into the hot skillet. Allow them to cook on each side for about five minutes. The thickness of the steak will determine how long you need to cook the steaks. Steaks that are a little over two inches should reach a medium cook in 5 minutes per side. If you prefer your steak more rare, cook for a shorter amount of time. For those who like a more well-done steak, cook for two minutes longer. Your steaks should have a nice brown color to them when they are done.

Once the steaks have reached your desired cook time, remove them from the skillet and place them on a plate, then cover them with aluminum foil to rest. Keep in mind your steaks will still continue to cook even though you have removed them from the skillet.

As the steaks rest, you want to make your sauce. Place a medium-sized saucepan on your stove and turn the heat to medium. Add in the butter and heavy cream. Once the butter has begun to melt, add in your spinach. Allow the spinach to cook down; this should only take about 5 minutes. Once the spinach has wilted, add in the parmesan cheese, sea salt, and black pepper. Stir, reduce heat to medium low and allow the sauce to thicken slightly for about 5 minutes.

Once the sauce is done, turn off the heat. Transfer your zucchini noodles to a large bowl and pour the sauce over top (leave a little sauce in the saucepan to top your steaks with). Toss the zucchini noodles with the sauce so that everything gets nicely coated. Add in the gorgonzola cheese, but reserve some to top your steaks with during plating. Toss everything one more time.

Now it is time to assemble the plate! Place a small portion of the zucchini noodles on your dinner plate, place a steak medallion on top of the noodles, and top with the dried tomatoes, gorgonzola crumbles, and a little drizzle of your leftover sauce.

Nutrition:

Calories 413

Carbs 6g

Fat 28g

Protein 30g

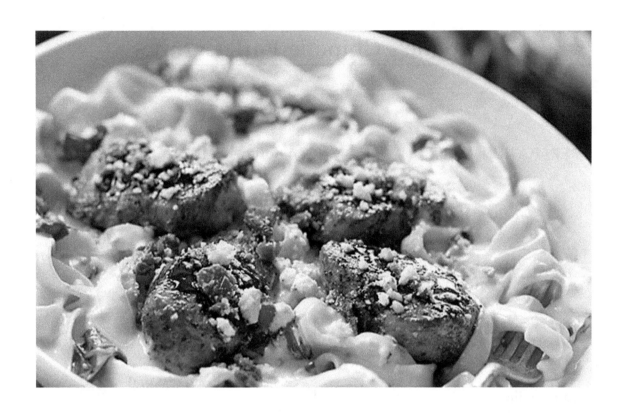

Chipotle's Chipotle Pork Carnitas

 PREPARATION: 5 MIN

 COOKING: 4 hours 10 MIN

 SERVING: 1/4

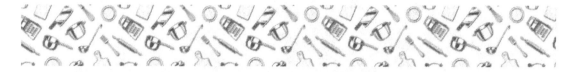

Ingredients:

1 cup water

2 tablespoons avocado oil

4 pounds pork roast

1 teaspoon thyme

2 teaspoon juniper berries

1 teaspoon Himalayan sea salt

½ teaspoon black pepper

Directions:

Begin by preheating your oven to 300 degrees Fahrenheit.

Next, take a Dutch oven pot, place it on your stove, and turn the heat to medium. Add the avocado oil to the pot.

As the pot heats, take your pork roast and sprinkle it with the sea salt. Then place the roast into the Dutch oven pot and brown the sides for a minute on each side.

Turn the heat off on the stove once the roast has browned. Add the water, thyme, juniper berries, and black pepper to the pot, then cover. Place the pot into your preheated oven and allow the roast to cook for 3 ½ hours. Turn the roast every half hour so that the flavors really penetrate into all areas of the meat.

Remove the roast from the oven after 3 ½ hours (keep the oven turned on), allow it to rest for 10 minutes, then use two forks to pull the meat apart. Once all the meat has been pulled, place the pot back into the oven for 30 minutes.

Remove the pot and enjoy!

Nutrition:

1. Calories 317
2. Carbs .5g
3. Fat 14.5g
4. Protein 43g

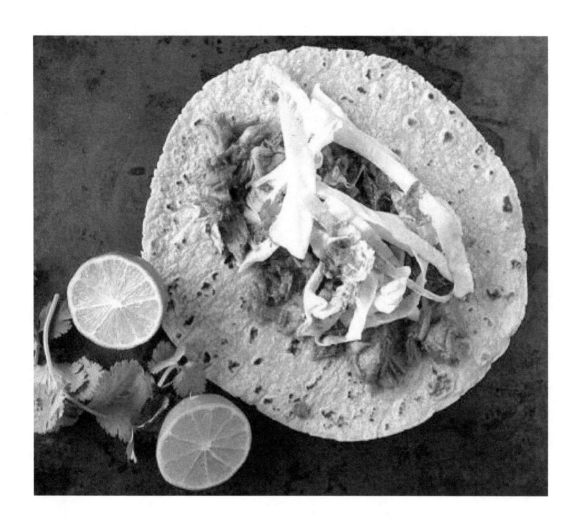

Chapter 4
Copycat Dessert Recipes

Chocolate Frosty - Wendy's

PREPARATION: 3 - 5 MIN

COOKING: 0 MIN

SERVING: 3

30 MIN freezing time

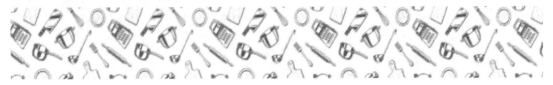

Ingredients:

heavy cream

unsweetened cocoa powder

Lakanto powdered sweetener

vanilla extract

Directions:

Collect heavy cream, unsweetened cocoa powder, Lakanto sweetener powder, and vanilla extract.

Mix the ingredients together in a big pot.

Mix until stiff peaks form; freeze for a minimum of 30 minutes.

To achieve the right consistency, either stir the mixture with a spoon or use a blender to soften the Frosty and give it the consistency not-completely-frozen / not-too-melty. Serve in a cup, a mug or a bottle and enjoy!

A spoonful of frosty keto chocolate being taken slightly out of the bowl.

Using Monkfruit Lakanto To Sweetener

In this recipe to Lakanto's Powdered Monkfruit was used and it turned out great and close to original! Monkfruit is a truly natural alternative sweetener, zero glycemic and tastes great! It works perfectly in almost any sweet recipe, and this Frosty keto chocolate is no exception. Powdered Monkfruit sweetener from Lakanto is a fantastic substitute for powdered sugar!

Nutrition:

1. Calories: 273.3
2. Fat: 32.3 g
3. Carbs: 4 g
4. Fibre: 1.3 g
5. Protein: 0.33 g
6. Net Carbs: 2.7g

Keto Cheesecake - Rocco

PREPARATION: 20 MIN

COOKING: 30 MIN

SERVING: 10 - 12

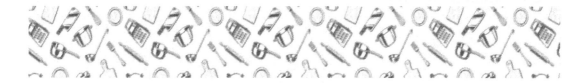

Ingredients:

Cream cheese or vegan cream cheese: 24 oz.

Yogurt: 2 cups such as yogurt of coconut milk

Pure vanilla extract: 2 1/2 tsp

Lemon juice: 1 tbsp. (optional)

Erythritol: 2/3 cup (sugar or maple syrup also work for non-keto)

Almond flour: 1/4 cup

Directions:

A crust store-bought can be used or render it crustless, or here's the crust used in recipe.2 cups of pecan flour or almond (pulse nuts can be used to create flour in a machine food processor) salt 1/4 tsp, melted coconut oil 4 to 6 tbsp. And sufficient water to render it sticky slightly.

All ingredients are combined, pour in an eight or nine-inch lined pan springform, evenly press down, and then set sideways while making the fill.

To 350 F oven is preheated. Fill the baking pan with water about halfway and on the lower rack of the oven place it. Let the cheese cream comes at room temperature, then all the ingredients are mixed in a food processor or blender till it is smooth (overbeating as it bakes can result in cracking). Typically lemon is added for a cheesecake flavor (classic), but leave it out if no one is there to give you hand, it will still work. Over the prepared crust top, the filling is spread. Place onto the middle rack (water pan is used above the rack). Bake for 30 min (or 38 min if an 8-inch pan is used), and during that time the oven should not be opened. Still don't open the oven once the time is completed, but the heat is turned off and the cheesecake is allowed in the oven for another 5 min. Now from the oven remove it — it will look still, Underdown. Now for 20 min allow it to be cooled on the counter, then overnight refrigerate it, and during the time it will significantly firm up. Important is cooling time so that the cake slowly cools down and therefore, it will not crack. Place the remains inside the refrigerator for 3 to 4 days, or freeze or you can slice it if needed.

Nutrition:

(Based On 12 Slices)

Calories 200

Total Fat 17 g

Saturated Fat 6.4 g

Cholesterol 0 mg

Sodium 240 mg

Total Carb 4 g

Net Carb 1.5 g

Dietary Fiber 2.5 g

Total Sugar 2 g

Added Sugar 0 g

Protein 4.5 g

Chapter 5
Copycat Soup Recipes

Pappadeaux's Crawfish Bisque

PREPARATION: 15 MIN

COOKING: 2 hours

SERVING: 1/4

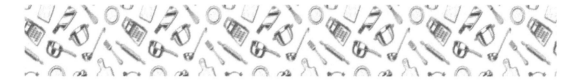

Ingredients:

4 cups water

1 tablespoon olive oil

1 ½ pounds of crawfish

¼ cup tomatoes (chopped)

¼ cup onions (chopped)

¼ cup green bell pepper (chopped)

1 ½ cups heavy cream

½ tablespoon tomato paste

½ teaspoon paprika

¼ teaspoon cayenne pepper

Directions:

Take a large pot filled with water and place it on your stove. Turn the heat to high to bring to a boil. Once the water is boiling, add your crawfish and boil for 15 minutes. Then turn off the heat and allow the crawfish to cool for 15 minutes.

Take the crawfish and separate the tail meat, set the shells and heads in a bowl to use for the stock later, and put the meat in a bowl to store in the refrigerator until you are ready for it.

Once you have separated the meat from the shells, place a large saucepan on your stove with the olive oil in it and turn the heat to medium heat. Add the heads and shells from the crawfish to the saucepan along with the cayenne pepper and paprika. Allow everything to sauté over medium heat for 5 minutes. Then, add the water and bring everything to a boil. Once the liquids are boiling, lower the heat to medium low and simmer for 30 minutes.

After 30 minutes, strain the liquid from the pan into a medium-sized bowl using a cheesecloth. Discard the shells and heads, then pour the liquid back into the saucepan. Turn the heat to medium low and add in the tomato paste, heavy cream, chopped tomatoes, onions, and green bell peppers. Allow the vegetables to simmer for 1 hour then add in the crawfish meat. Simmer everything for another 15 minutes then serve.

Nutrition:

Calories 275

Carbs 2.5g

Fat 18g

Protein 25g

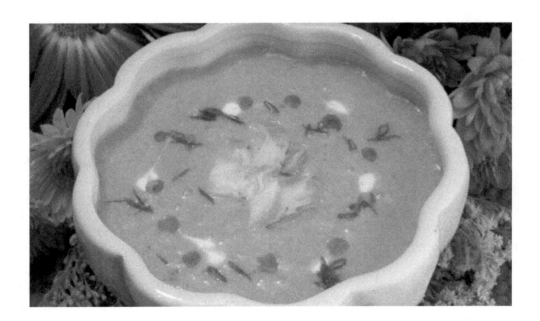

Panera Bread's Broccoli Cheddar Soup

PREPARATION: 10 MIN

COOKING: 25 MIN

SERVING: 1/6

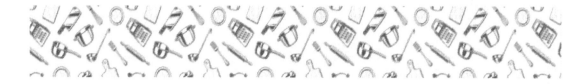

Ingredients:

1 tablespoon olive oil

3 ½ cups low-sodium chicken or vegetable broth

½ cup heavy cream

2 cups broccoli (chopped)

1 cup carrots (shredded)

½ cup white onions (diced fine)

4 ounces of cheddar cheese (shredded)

4 ounces gouda cheese

4 ounces cream cheese

¼ teaspoon black pepper

Directions:

Get a large saucepan and place it on your stovetop. Add the olive oil to the pan and turn the heat to medium. Allow the pan to heat for a few minutes then add your onions and sauté them for about 5 minutes.

Add the cream cheese to the pan and stir frequently to allow the cheese to begin to melt. Slowly pour in the heavy cream, then add in the gouda and shredded cheddar cheese. Continue to stir for 3 minutes.

Add your chopped broccoli to the pan along with the chicken or vegetable broth. Allow the broth to simmer for 5 minutes, then add in the carrots and black pepper. Lower the heat to medium low, cover, and let the soup cook for 10 minutes.

After 10 minutes, you can take half the soup and transfer it to a blender. Blend on high until you have a smooth consistency, then transfer back into the pan and stir until everything comes together. This will give you a slightly thicker but smoother soup. If you want a chunkier soup, then just serve hot after it has cooked for 10 minutes in the step before.

Nutrition:

Calories 295

Carbs 5g

Fat 24g

Protein 13g

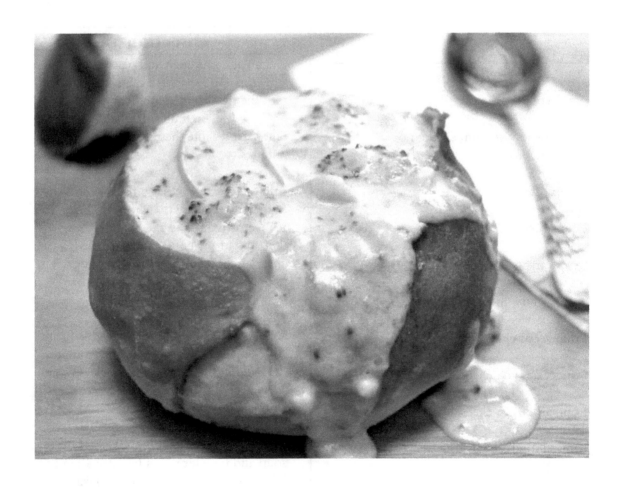

Chapter 6
Copycat and Dressing Recipes

Olive Garden Three Meat Sauce

PREPARATION: 15 MIN

COOKING: 40 MIN

SERVING: 8

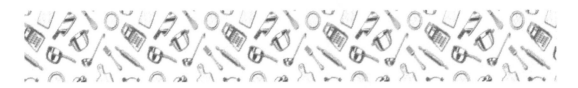

Ingredients:

½ pound ground beef

½ pound Italian sausage, casing removed

2 tablespoons olive oil

1 cup onions, chopped

24 ounces sugar-free marinara sauce

1 (16-ounce) can crushed tomatoes

¼ cup pepperoni, chopped finely

1 teaspoon Italian seasonings

Salt and ground black pepper, as required

Directions:

Heat a large skillet over medium-high heat and cook the beef and sausage for about 8-10 minutes or until done completely,

Meanwhile, in a large saucepan, heat the oil over medium heat and sauté the onion for about 4-5 minutes.

Add the marina sauce, tomatoes, and stir to combine.

Drain the grease from skillet of meat and transfer into the pan of sauce and stir to combine well.

In the pan, add the pepperoni and Italian seasonings and stir to combine.

Reduce the heat to low and simmer for about 20-25 minutes, stirring occasionally.

Stir in the salt and black pepper and remove from the heat.

Serve hot.

Tip:

Make sure to use sugar-free marinara sauce.

Nutrition:

1. Calories: 267Kcal;
2. Proteins: 16.5g;
3. Carbohydrates: 10g;
4. Fat: 17.7g

Olive Garden Spinach Alfredo Sauce

PREPARATION: 15 MIN   **COOKING: 16 MIN**   **SERVING: 5**

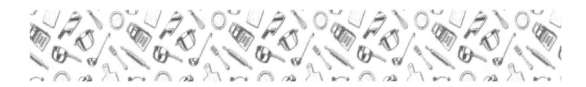

Ingredients

½ cup butter

¾ cup frozen chopped spinach, thawed

2 cups heavy whipping cream

3 tablespoons cream cheese

1 cup Parmesan cheese, grated

1 teaspoon garlic powder

Salt and ground black pepper, as required

Directions

In a pan, melt butter over low heat and cook the spinach for about 1 minute.

Stir in the cream and cream cheese and cook for about 5 minutes, stirring continuously.

Stir in the Parmesan cheese, garlic powder, salt, and black pepper and cook for about 10 minutes.

Tip:

Microwave the frozen spinach for 1-2 minutes to thaw completely.

Nutrition

Calories: 44Kcal;

Proteins: 21g;

Carbohydrates: 5.3g;

Fat: 51.1g

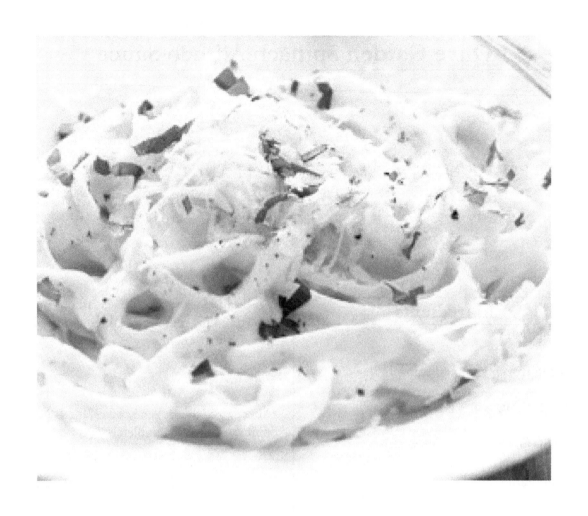

Chapter 7
Smoothies Recipes

Peanut Butter Cup Smoothie

PREPARATION: 5 MIN   **COOKING: 0 MIN**   **SERVING: 2**

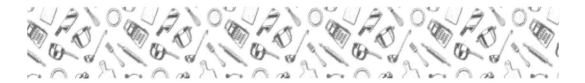

Ingredients

1 cup water

¾ cup coconut cream

1 scoop chocolate protein powder

2 tablespoons natural peanut butter

3 ice cubes

Directions

Put the water, coconut cream, protein powder, peanut butter, and ice in a blender and blend until smooth.

Pour into 2 glasses and serve immediately.

Nutrition

Calories: 486

Fat: 40g

Protein: 30g

Carbs: 11g

Fiber: 5g

Net Carbs: 6g

Berry Green Smoothie

PREPARATION: 10 MIN   **COOKING: 0 MIN**   **SERVING: 2**

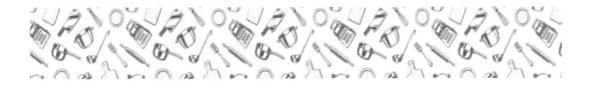

Ingredients

1 cup water

½ cup raspberries

½ cup shredded kale

¾ cup cream cheese

1 tablespoon coconut oil

1 scoop vanilla protein powder

Directions

Put the water, raspberries, kale, cream cheese, coconut oil, and protein powder in a blender and blend until smooth.

Pour into 2 glasses and serve immediately.

Nutrition

Calories: 436

Fat: 36g

Protein: 28g

Carbs: 11g

Fiber: 5g

Net Carbs: 6g

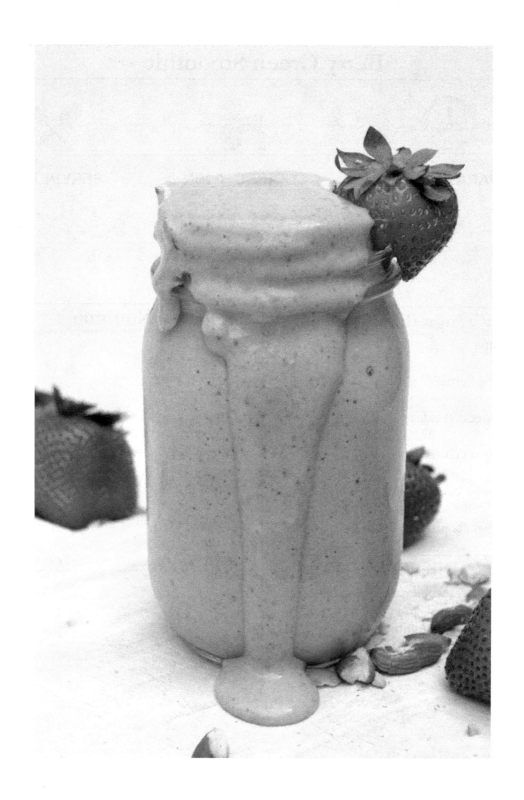

Chapter 8
Keto Side Dishes and Snacks

Roasted Cauliflower With Prosciutto, Capers, And Almonds

PREPARATION: 5 MIN

COOKING: 25 MIN

SERVING: 2

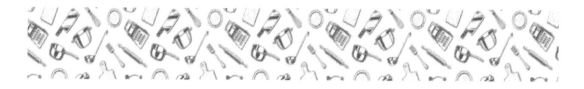

Ingredients

12 ounces cauliflower florets (I get precut florets at Trader Joe's)

2 tablespoons leftover bacon grease, or olive oil

Pink Himalayan salt

Freshly ground black pepper

2 ounces sliced prosciutto, torn into small pieces

¼ cup slivered almonds

2 tablespoons capers

2 tablespoons grated Parmesan cheese

Directions

Preheat the oven to 400°F. Line a baking pan with a silicone baking mat or parchment paper.

Put the cauliflower florets in the prepared baking pan with the bacon grease, and season with pink Himalayan salt and pepper. Or if you are using olive oil instead, drizzle the cauliflower with olive oil and season with pink Himalayan salt and pepper.

Roast the cauliflower for 15 minutes.

Stir the cauliflower so all sides are coated with the bacon grease.

Distribute the prosciutto pieces in the pan. Then add the slivered almonds and capers. Stir to combine. Sprinkle the Parmesan cheese on top, and roast for 10 minutes more.

Divide between two plates, using a slotted spoon so you don't get excess grease in the plates, and serve.

SUBSTITUTION TIP Sliced green olives work well if you don't have capers.

Nutrition

1. Calories: 288;
2. Total Fat: 24g;
3. Carbs: 7g;
4. Net Carbs: 4g;
5. Fiber: 3g;
6. Protein: 14g

Buttery Slow-Cooker Mushrooms

PREPARATION: 10 MIN

COOKING: 4 hours

SERVING: 2

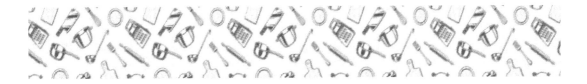

Ingredients:

6 tablespoons butter

1 tablespoon packaged dry ranch-dressing mix

8 ounces fresh cremini mushrooms

2 tablespoons grated Parmesan cheese

1 tablespoon chopped fresh flat-leaf Italian parsley

Directions:

With the crock insert in place, preheat the slow cooker to low.

Put the butter and the dry ranch dressing in the bottom of the slow cooker, and allow the butter to melt. Stir to blend the dressing mix and butter.

Add the mushrooms to the slow cooker, and stir to coat with the butter-dressing mixture. Sprinkle the top with the Parmesan cheese.

Cover and cook on low for 4 hours.

Use a slotted spoon to transfer the mushrooms to a serving dish. Top with the chopped parsley and serve.

SUBSTITUTION TIP If you don't have dry ranch-dressing mix, for a similar result you can combine equal amounts of onion powder, garlic powder, dried thyme, pink Himalayan salt, pepper, dried parsley, and a dash of paprika.

Nutrition:

1. Calories: 351;
2. Total Fat: 36g;
3. Carbs: 5g;
4. Net Carbs: 4g;
5. Fiber: 1g;
6. Protein: 6g

Baked Zucchini Gratin

PREPARATION: 10 MIN,

COOKING: 25 MIN

SERVING: 2

30 MIN to drain

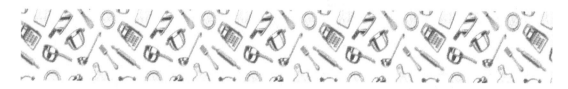

Ingredients

1 large zucchini, cut into ¼-inch-thick slices

Pink Himalayan salt

1 ounce Brie cheese, rind trimmed off

1 tablespoon butter

Freshly ground black pepper

1/3 cup shredded Gruyère cheese

¼ cup crushed pork rinds

Directions

Salt the zucchini slices and put them in a colander in the sink for 45 minutes; the zucchini will shed much of their water.

Preheat the oven to 400°F.

When the zucchini have been "weeping" for about 30 minutes, in a small saucepan over medium-low heat, heat the Brie and butter, stirring occasionally, until the cheese has melted and the mixture is fully combined, about 2 minutes.

Arrange the zucchini in an 8-inch baking dish so the zucchini slices are overlapping a bit. Season with pepper.

Pour the Brie mixture over the zucchini, and top with the shredded Gruyère cheese.

Sprinkle the crushed pork rinds over the top.

Bake for about 25 minutes, until the dish is bubbling and the top is nicely browned, and serve.

SUBSTITUTION TIP You can use a crème de Brie soft cheese as well. Some have garlic or other herbs in

them, which are tasty additions to this dish.

Nutrition

Calories: 355;

Total Fat: 25g;

Carbs: 5g;

Net Carbs: 4g;

Fiber: 2g;

Protein: 28g

Roasted Radishes With Brown Butter Sauce

PREPARATION: 10 MIN

COOKING: 15 MIN

SERVING: 2

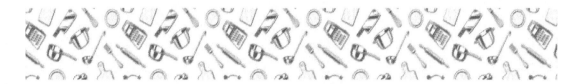

Ingredients:

2 cups halved radishes

1 tablespoon olive oil

Pink Himalayan salt

Freshly ground black pepper

2 tablespoons butter

1 tablespoon chopped fresh flat-leaf Italian parsley

Directions:

Preheat the oven to 450°F.

In a medium bowl, toss the radishes in the olive oil and season with pink Himalayan salt and pepper.

Spread the radishes on a baking sheet in a single layer. Roast for 15 minutes, stirring halfway through.

Meanwhile, when the radishes have been roasting for about 10 minutes, in a small, light-colored saucepan over medium heat, melt the butter completely, stirring frequently, and season with pink Himalayan salt. When the butter begins to bubble and foam, continue stirring. When the bubbling diminishes a bit, the butter should be a nice nutty brown. The browning process should take about 3 minutes total. Transfer the browned butter to a heat-safe container (I use a mug).

Remove the radishes from the oven, and divide them between two plates. Spoon the brown butter over the radishes, top with the chopped parsley, and serve.

INGREDIENT TIP You can keep the stems on the radishes to roast them if you prefer them that way.

Nutrition:

Calories: 181;

Total Fat: 19g;

Carbs: 4g;

Net Carbs: 2g;

Fiber: 2g;

Protein: 1g

Parmesan And Pork Rind Green Beans

PREPARATION: 5 MIN

COOKING: 15 MIN

SERVING: 2

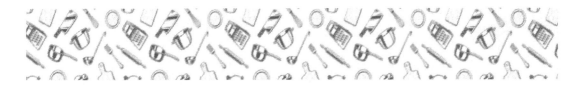

Ingredients:

½ pound fresh green beans

2 tablespoons crushed pork rinds

2 tablespoons olive oil

1 tablespoon grated Parmesan cheese

Pink Himalayan salt

Freshly ground black pepper

Directions:

Preheat the oven to 400°F.

In a medium bowl, combine the green beans, pork rinds, olive oil, and Parmesan cheese. Season with pink Himalayan salt and pepper, and toss until the beans are thoroughly coated.

Spread the bean mixture on a baking sheet in a single layer, and roast for about 15 minutes. At the halfway point, give the pan a little shake to move the beans around, or just give them a stir.

Divide the beans between two plates and serve.

INGREDIENT TIP You can use any flavor of pork rinds to add additional zest to the green beans, but I typically use the original flavor.

Nutrition:

Calories: 175;

Total Fat: 15g;

Carbs: 8g;

Net Carbs: 5g;

Fiber: 3g;

Protein: 6g

Chapter 9
Keto Pasta Recipes

Creamy Zoodles

PREPARATION: 2 MIN

COOKING: 3 MIN

SERVING: 1

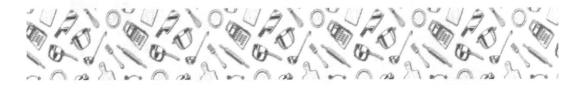

Ingredients

Three (3) cloves of minced garlic

Two (2) tablespoons of butter

Two (2) medium zucchini

A quarter teaspoon salt to taste

A quarter teaspoon pepper

A quarter cup of parmesan cheese

Directions

Wash your zucchini then cut it to strands using a spiralizer or vegetable peeler then set aside. If done right, your zucchini should come out like spaghetti strands. I mean, that's the point right?

Put a large pan on medium heat. Put the butter in to melt and then add minced garlic. Stir fry the garlic until it starts to appear translucent. If you know you have an affinity for burning things, please be attentive so the garlic doesn't get burnt.

Add your zucchini strands and stir fry for three minutes. Make sure to taste your noodle strands to check how tender they are as zucchini cooks really fast. Try not to "taste" till it finishes.

Bring down the pan, add salt, pepper and parmesan cheese, stir until well combined and serve..

Nutrition

Calories: 100

Total Fat: 4g

Carbs: 4g

Protein: 4g

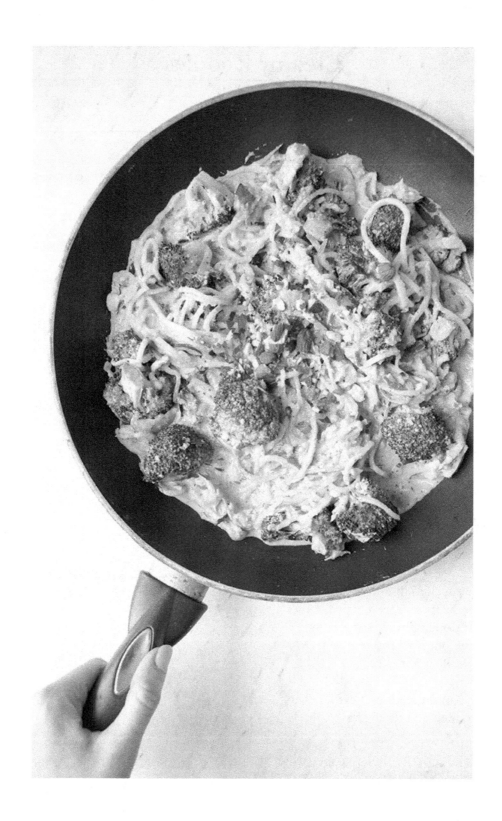

Keto Carbonara Pasta

PREPARATION: 10 MIN

COOKING: 15 MIN

SERVING: 1

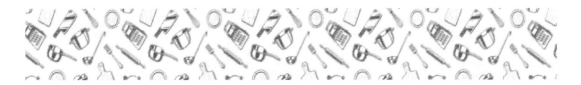

Ingredients

150 grams of bacon

One large egg yolk

A packet of miracle noodles

A cup of heavy whipping cream

Two (2) tablespoons of parmesan cheese

60 grams of chicken breast

Directions

Dice the chicken and Chicken in separate plates.

Set both to cook separately in a frying pan for 5 minutes.

Note: Do not let the bacon become crispy.

Put parmesan cheese and egg yolk in a small bowl and mix until it forms a paste.

Pour the cheese mixture into a frying pan and put on medium heat.

Add half the amount of cream and mix until a smooth creamy paste is formed.

Add the other half of the cream, bacon and chicken. Stir until fully coated.

Dry fry miracle noodles in another pan for 10 minutes, stirring continuously so it doesn't stick or burn.

Mix the noodles with sauce and serve.

Nutrition

1. Calories: 580
2. Total Fat: 50g
3. Carbs: 5g
4. Protein: 27g

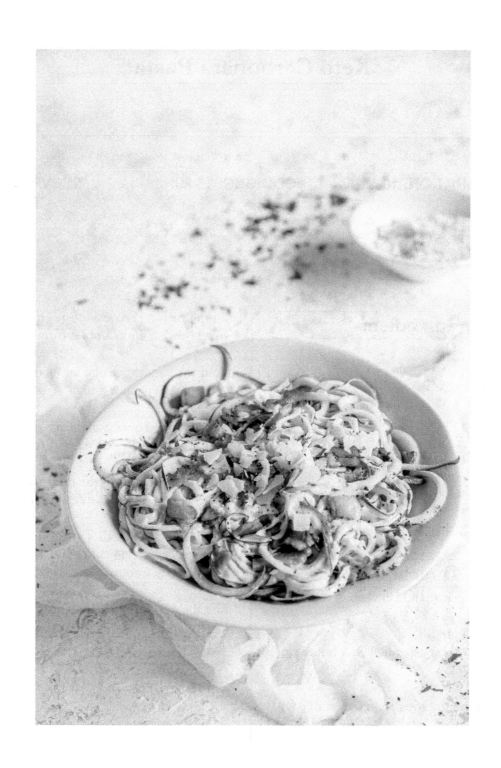

Chapter 10
More Keto Recipes

Nut Medley Granola

PREPARATION: 10 MIN **COOKING: 1 hour** **SERVING: 8**

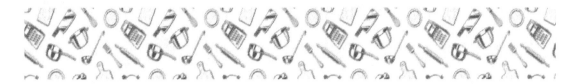

Ingredients

2 cups shredded unsweetened coconut

1 cup sliced almonds

1 cup raw sunflower seeds

½ cup raw pumpkin seeds

½ cup walnuts

½ cup melted coconut oil

10 drops liquid stevia

1 teaspoon ground cinnamon

½ teaspoon ground nutmeg

Directions:

Preheat the oven to 250°F. Line 2 baking sheets with parchment paper. Set aside.

Toss together the shredded coconut, almonds, sunflower seeds, pumpkin seeds, and walnuts in a large bowl until mixed.

In a small bowl, stir together the coconut oil, stevia, cinnamon, and nutmeg until blended.

Pour the coconut oil mixture into the nut mixture and use your hands to blend until the nuts are very well coated.

Transfer the granola mixture to the baking sheets and spread it out evenly.

Bake the granola, stirring every 10 to 15 minutes, until the mixture is golden brown and crunchy, about 1 hour.

Transfer the granola to a large bowl and let the granola cool, tossing it frequently to break up the large pieces.

Store the granola in airtight containers in the refrigerator or freezer for up to 1 month.

Nutrition

Calories: 391

Fat: 38g

Protein: 10g

Carbs: 10g

Fiber: 6g

Net Carbs: 4g

Bacon-Artichoke Omelet

PREPARATION: 10 MIN   **COOKING: 10 MIN**   **SERVING: 4**

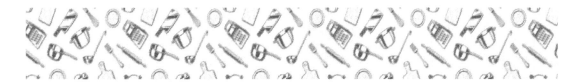

Ingredients

6 eggs, beaten

2 tablespoons heavy (whipping) cream

8 bacon slices, cooked and chopped

1 tablespoon olive oil

¼ cup chopped onion

½ cup chopped artichoke hearts (canned, packed in water)

Sea salt

Freshly ground black pepper

Directions

In a small bowl, whisk together the eggs, heavy cream, and bacon until well blended, and set aside.

Place a large skillet over medium-high heat and add the olive oil.

Sauté the onion until tender, about 3 minutes.

Pour the egg mixture into the skillet, swirling it for 1 minute.

Cook the omelet, lifting the edges with a spatula to let the uncooked egg flow underneath, for 2 minutes.

Sprinkle the artichoke hearts on top and flip the omelet. Cook for 4 minutes more, until the egg is firm. Flip the omelet over again so the artichoke hearts are on top.

Remove from the heat, cut the omelet into quarters, and season with salt and black pepper. Transfer the omelet to plates and serve.

Nutrition

Calories: 435

Fat: 39g

Protein: 17g

Carbs: 5g

Fiber: 2g

Net Carbs: 3g

Mushroom Frittata

PREPARATION: 10 MIN **COOKING: 15 MIN** **SERVING: 6**

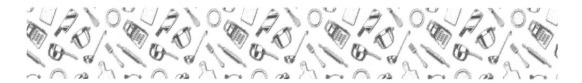

Ingredients

2 tablespoons olive oil

1 cup sliced fresh mushrooms

1 cup shredded spinach

6 bacon slices, cooked and chopped

10 large eggs, beaten

½ cup crumbled goat cheese

Sea salt

Freshly ground black pepper

Directions:

Preheat the oven to 350°F.

Place a large ovenproof skillet over medium-high heat and add the olive oil.

Sauté the mushrooms until lightly browned, about 3 minutes.

Add the spinach and bacon and sauté until the greens are wilted, about 1 minute.

Add the eggs and cook, lifting the edges of the frittata with a spatula so uncooked egg flows underneath, for 3 to 4 minutes.

Sprinkle the top with the crumbled goat cheese and season lightly with salt and pepper.

Bake until set and lightly browned, about 15 minutes.

Remove the frittata from the oven, and let it stand for 5 minutes.

Cut into 6 wedges and serve immediately.

SUBSTITUTION TIP If you're not keen on goat cheese, feta cheese tastes lovely with the other ingredients in this dish. Feta is higher in fat and lower in protein than goat cheese, so keep that in mind when considering your keto macros.

Nutrition

Calories: 316

Fat: 27g

Protein: 16g

Carbs: 1g

Fiber: 0g

Net Carbs: 1g

Breakfast Bake

PREPARATION: 10 MIN

COOKING: 50 MIN

SERVING: 8

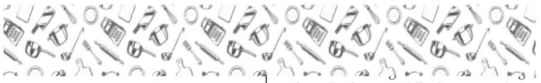

Ingredients

1 tablespoon olive oil, plus extra for greasing the casserole dish

1 pound preservative-free or homemade sausage

8 large eggs

2 cups cooked spaghetti squash

1 tablespoon chopped fresh oregano

Sea salt

Freshly ground black pepper

½ cup shredded Cheddar cheese

Directions

Preheat the oven to 375°F. Lightly grease a 9-by-13-inch casserole dish with olive oil and set aside.

Place a large ovenproof skillet over medium-high heat and add the olive oil.

about 5 minutes. While the sausage is cooking, whisk together the eggs, squash, and oregano in a medium bowl. Season lightly with salt and pepper and set aside.

Add the cooked sausage to the egg mixture, stir until just combined, and pour the mixture into the casserole dish.

Sprinkle the top of the casserole with the cheese and cover the casserole loosely with aluminum foil.

Bake the casserole for 30 minutes, and then remove the foil and bake for an additional 15 minutes.

Let the casserole stand for 10 minutes before serving.

Nutrition

1. Calories: 303
2. Fat: 24g
3. Protein: 17g
4. Carbs: 4g
5. Fiber: 1g
6. Net Carbs: 3g

Avocado And Eggs

PREPARATION: 10 MIN

COOKING: 20 MIN

SERVING: 4

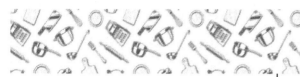

Ingredients

2 avocados, peeled, halved lengthwise, and pitted

4 large eggs

1 (4-ounce) chicken breast, cooked and shredded

¼ cup Cheddar cheese

Sea salt

Freshly ground black pepper

Directions:

Preheat the oven to 425°F.

Take a spoon and hollow out each side of the avocado halves until the hole is about twice the original size.

Place the avocado halves in an 8-by-8-inch baking dish, hollow-side up.

[...] shredded chicken between each avocado half. Sprinkle the cheese on top of each and season lightly with the salt and pepper.

Bake the avocados until the eggs are cooked through, about 15 to 20 minutes.

Serve immediately.

PREP TIP Cooked chicken breast is very handy for many recipes, so bake 4 or 5 breasts at the beginning of the week and store them in a sealed plastic bag in the refrigerator after they are completely cooled. Cooked chicken will keep for up to 5 days in the refrigerator.

Nutrition

Calories: 324

Fat: 25g

Protein: 19g

Carbs: 8g

Fiber: 5g

Net Carbs: 3g

Cheesy Garden Veggie Crustless Quiche

PREPARATION: 5 MIN

COOKING: 25 MIN

SERVING: 4

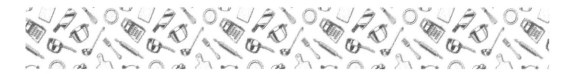

Ingredients

1 tablespoon grass-fed butter, divided

6 eggs

¾ cup heavy (whipping) cream

3 ounces goat cheese, divided

½ cup sliced mushrooms, chopped

1 scallion, white and green parts, chopped

1 cup shredded fresh spinach

10 cherry tomatoes, cut in half

Directions:

Preheat the oven. Set the oven temperature to 350°F. Grease a 9-inch pie plate with ½ teaspoon of the butter and set it aside.

Mix the quiche base. In a medium bowl, whisk the eggs, cream, and 2 ounces of the cheese until it's all well blended. Set it aside.

Sauté the vegetables. In a small skillet over medium-high heat, melt the remaining butter. Add the mushrooms and scallion and sauté them until they've softened, about 2 minutes. Add the spinach and sauté until it's wilted, about 2 minutes.

Assemble and bake. Spread the vegetable mixture in the bottom of the pie plate and pour the egg-and-cream mixture over the vegetables. Scatter the cherry tomatoes and the remaining 1 ounce of goat cheese on top. Bake for 20 to 25 minutes until the quiche is cooked through, puffed, and lightly browned.

Serve. Cut the quiche into wedges and divide it between four plates. Serve it warm or cold.

Tip: You can bake this in muffin tins as well if handy, grab-and-go quiches work better for you. Grease the cups of a 6-cup muffin tin, divide the vegetable mixture between them, and pour in the egg mixture. Bake them for 12 to 15 minutes. This will not change the macros, but your calories will be 237 per "muffin."

Nutrition:

Macronutrients: Fat: 75%; Protein: 20%; Carbs: 5%

Calories: 355; Total fat: 30g; Total carbs: 5g; Fiber: 1g;

Net carbs: 4g; Sodium: 228mg; Protein: 18g

Zucchini Roll Manicotti

PREPARATION: 15 MIN   **COOKING: 30 MIN**   **SERVING: 4**

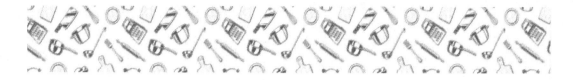

Ingredients:

Olive oil cooking spray

4 zucchini

2 tablespoons good-quality olive oil

1 red bell pepper, diced

½ onion, minced

2 teaspoons minced garlic

1 cup goat cheese

1 cup shredded mozzarella cheese

1 tablespoon chopped fresh oregano

Sea salt, for seasoning

Freshly ground black pepper, for seasoning

2 cups low-carb marinara sauce, divided

½ cup grated Parmesan cheese

Directions:

Preheat the oven. Set the oven temperature to 375°F. Lightly grease a 9-by-13-inch baking dish with olive oil cooking spray.

Prepare the zucchini. Cut the zucchini lengthwise into 1/8-inch-thick slices and set them aside.

Make the filling. In a medium skillet over medium-high heat, warm the olive oil. Add the red bell pepper, onion, and garlic and sauté until they've softened, about 4 minutes. Remove the skillet from the heat and transfer the vegetables to a medium bowl. Stir the goat cheese, mozzarella, and oregano into the vegetables. Season it all with salt and pepper.

Assemble the manicotti. Spread 1 cup of the marinara sauce in the bottom of the baking dish. Lay a zucchini slice on a clean cutting board and place a couple tablespoons of filling at one end. Roll the slice up and place it in the baking dish, seam-side down. Repeat with the remaining zucchini slices. Spoon the remaining sauce over the rolls and top with the Parmesan.

Bake. Bake the rolls for 30 to 35 minutes until the zucchini is tender and the cheese is golden.

Serve. Spoon the rolls onto four plates and serve them hot.

Tip: If you have time, you can lightly blanch the zucchini slices and drain them before rolling so that the casserole has less liquid in it from the juices and the slices roll easily. To blanch: Dunk the zucchini slices in boiling water. Leave them there for about 3 minutes, then remove them and run them under cold water or put them in a bowl filled with ice water for a few minutes to stop them from cooking any more.

Nutrition:

Macronutrients: Fat: 63%; Protein: 14%; Carbs: 23%

Calories: 342; Total fat: 24g; Total carbs: 14g; Fiber: 3g;

Net carbs: 11g; Sodium: 331mg; Protein: 20g

Spinach Artichoke Stuffed Peppers

PREPARATION: 10 MIN

COOKING: 20 MIN

SERVING: 4

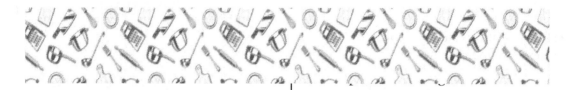

Ingredients:

4 red bell peppers, halved and seeded

1 tablespoon good-quality olive oil, for drizzling

Sea salt, for seasoning

Freshly ground black pepper, for seasoning

2 cups finely chopped cauliflower

10 ounces chopped fresh spinach

2 cups chopped marinated artichoke hearts

1 cup cream cheese, softened

1½ cups shredded mozzarella cheese, divided

½ cup sour cream

2 tablespoons mayonnaise

Directions:

Preheat the oven. Set the oven temperature to 400°F. Line a baking sheet with parchment paper.

Prepare the peppers. Place the red bell peppers cut-side up on the baking sheet. Lightly grease them all over with the olive oil and season them with salt and pepper.

Make the filling. In a large bowl, mix together the cauliflower, spinach, artichoke hearts, cream cheese, ¾ cup of the mozzarella, and the sour cream, mayonnaise, and garlic.

Stuff and bake. Stuff the peppers with the filling and sprinkle with the remaining ¾ cup of mozzarella. Bake them for 20 to 25 minutes until the filling is heated through, bubbly, and lightly browned.

Serve. Place one stuffed pepper on each of four plates and serve them hot.

Swap: Use goat cheese instead of cream cheese and thick Greek-style yogurt instead of sour cream for a satisfying tangy flavor and velvety texture. This swap will change the macros to Fat: 62%; Protein: 26%; Carbs: 12%.

Nutrition:

Macronutrients: Fat: 72%; Protein: 16%; Carbs: 12%

Calories: 523; Total fat: 43g; Total carbs: 19g; Fiber: 7g;

Net carbs: 12g; Sodium: 355mg; Protein: 19g

Zucchini Pasta With Spinach, Olives, And Asiago

PREPARATION: 10 MIN

COOKING: 10 MIN

SERVING: 4

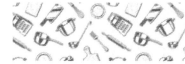

Ingredients:

3 tablespoons good-quality olive oil

1 tablespoon grass-fed butter

1½ tablespoons minced garlic

1 cup packed fresh spinach

½ cup sliced black olives

½ cup halved cherry tomatoes

2 tablespoons chopped fresh basil

3 zucchini, spiralized

Sea salt, for seasoning

Freshly ground black pepper, for seasoning

½ cup shredded Asiago cheese

Directions:

Sauté the vegetables. In a large skillet over medium-high heat, warm the olive oil and butter. Add the garlic and sauté until it's tender, about 2 minutes. Stir in the spinach, olives, tomatoes, and basil and sauté until the spinach is wilted, about 4 minutes. Stir in the zucchini noodles, toss to combine them with the sauce, and cook until the zucchini is tender, about 2 minutes.

Serve. Season with salt and pepper. Divide the mixture between four bowls and serve topped with the Asiago.

Tip: To save time, spiralize the zucchini ahead and store it in a sealed container in the fridge for up to three days, or buy it pre-spiralized.

Nutrition:

Macronutrients: Fat: 80%; Protein: 13%; Carbs: 7%

Calories: 199; Total fat: 18g; Total carbs: 4g; Fiber: 1g;

Net carbs: 3g; Sodium: 363mg; Protein: 6g

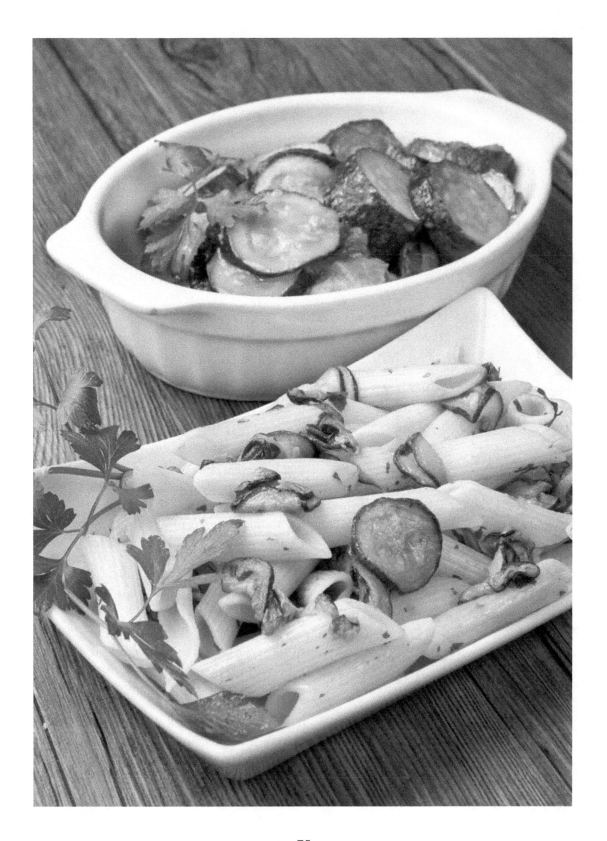

Vegetable Vodka Sauce Bake

PREPARATION: 10 MIN

COOKING: 30 MIN

SERVING: 4

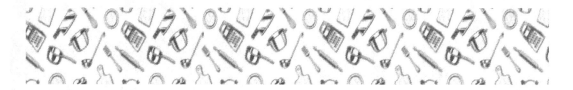

Ingredients:

3 tablespoons melted grass-fed butter, divided

4 cups mushrooms, halved

4 cups cooked cauliflower florets

1½ cups purchased vodka sauce (see Tip)

¾ cup heavy (whipping) cream

½ cup grated Asiago cheese

Sea salt, for seasoning

Freshly ground black pepper, for seasoning

1 cup shredded provolone cheese

2 tablespoons chopped fresh oregano

Directions:

Preheat the oven. Set the oven temperature to 350°F and use 1 tablespoon of the melted butter to grease a 9-by-13-inch baking dish.

Mix the vegetables. In a large bowl, combine the mushrooms, cauliflower, vodka sauce, cream, Asiago, and the remaining 2 tablespoons of butter. Season the vegetables with salt and pepper.

Bake. Transfer the vegetable mixture to the baking dish and top it with the provolone cheese. Bake for 30 to 35 minutes until it's bubbly and heated through.

Serve. Divide the mixture between four plates and top with the oregano.

Tip: You can make your own vodka sauce if you have a favorite recipe, but there are many very good ones at the store that save time and money, which is why that's what I recommend here. Just be sure you're choosing one without any added sugar (or if you're making it from scratch, skip any recipe step that includes sugar).

Nutrition:

Macronutrients: Fat: 75%; Protein: 10%; Carbs: 15%

Calories: 537; Total fat: 45g; Total carbs: 14g; Fiber: 6g;

Net carbs: 8g; Sodium: 527mg; Protein: 19g

Greek Vegetable Briam

PREPARATION: 10 MIN   **COOKING: 30 MIN**   **SERVING: 4**

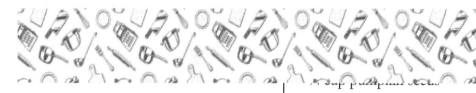

Ingredients:

1/3 cup good-quality olive oil, divided

1 onion, thinly sliced

1 tablespoon minced garlic

¾ small eggplant, diced

2 zucchini, diced

2 cups chopped cauliflower

1 red bell pepper, diced

2 cups diced tomatoes

2 tablespoons chopped fresh parsley

2 tablespoons chopped fresh oregano

Sea salt, for seasoning

Freshly ground black pepper, for seasoning

1½ cups crumbled feta cheese

Directions:

Preheat the oven. Set the oven to broil and lightly grease a 9-by-13-inch casserole dish with olive oil.

Sauté the aromatics. In a medium stockpot over medium heat, warm 3 tablespoons of the olive oil. Add the onion and garlic and sauté until they've softened, about 3 minutes.

Sauté the vegetables. Stir in the eggplant and cook for 5 minutes, stirring occasionally. Add the zucchini, cauliflower, and red bell pepper and cook for 5 minutes. Stir in the tomatoes, parsley, and oregano and cook, giving it a stir from time to time, until the vegetables are tender, about 10 minutes. Season it with salt and pepper.

Broil. Transfer the vegetable mixture to the casserole dish and top with the crumbled feta. Broil for about 4 minutes until the cheese is golden.

Serve. Divide the casserole between four plates and top it with the pumpkin seeds. Drizzle with the remaining olive oil.

Tip: This is a great dish to make ahead. Follow the recipe right up until it's ready to go under the broiler. Cover the casserole dish with aluminum foil and refrigerate for up to two days. To reheat, remove the foil and pop it in the oven at 375°F for a delicious meal in 20 minutes.

Make sure you still broil it for a few minutes to create a golden top.

Nutrition:

Macronutrients: Fat: 70%; Protein: 11%; Carbs: 19%

Calories: 356; Total fat: 28g; Total carbs: 18g; Fiber: 7g;

Net carbs: 11g; Sodium: 467mg; Protein: 11g

Flappa Jacks

PREPARATION: 10 MIN　　**COOKING: 14 MIN**　　**SERVING:**

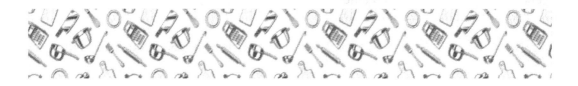

Ingredients:

1 cup blanched almond flour

¼ cup coconut flour

5 large eggs, whisked

3 (1-gram) packets 0g net carb sweetener

1 teaspoon baking powder

1/3 cup unsweetened almond milk

¼ cup vegetable oil

1½ teaspoons pure vanilla extract

1/8 teaspoon salt

Directions:

In a large mixing bowl, mix all ingredients together until smooth.

In a large nonstick skillet over medium heat, pour desired-sized pancakes and cook 3–5 minutes until bubbles form.

Flip pancakes and cook another 2 minutes until brown. Repeat as needed to use all batter. Serve.

Nutrition:

Calories 273

Fat 23g

Protein 10g

Sodium 202mg

Fiber 4g

Carbohydrates 7g

Sugar 2g

Booga Chia Cereal

PREPARATION: 2 MIN+　　　**COOKING: 0 MIN**　　　**SERVING:**

Refrigeration Overnight

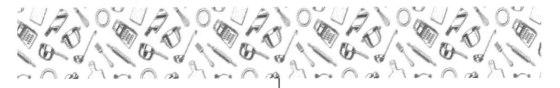

Ingredients:

2 tablespoons chia seeds

2 (1-gram) packets 0g net carb sweetener

½ cup unsweetened almond milk

1/8 teaspoon pure vanilla extract

Directions:

Add all ingredients to a small container or bowl. Stir until blended.

Let soak overnight in refrigerator for best results as chia seeds soften as they absorb liquid and swell.

Serve the next morning.

Nutrition:

Calories 132

Fat 9g

Protein 4g

Sodium 93mg

Fiber 9g

Carbohydrates 11g

Sugar 0g

Sawdust Oatmeal

PREPARATION: 5 MIN

COOKING: 0 MIN

SERVING:

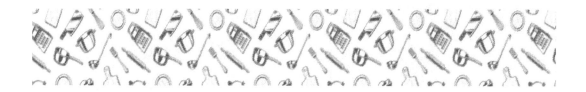

Ingredients:

1/3 cup boiling water

2 tablespoons chia seeds

2 tablespoons flaxseed meal

2 tablespoons heavy whipping cream

1 (1-gram) packet 0g net carb sweetener

Directions:

Add all ingredients to a small glass or porcelain bowl. Stir to mix. Be careful as water is very hot.

Stir every couple of minutes as it cools to ensure even cooling. The chia seeds soften and expand as they absorb liquid.

When it's cool, it's ready to eat.

Nutrition:

Calories   289

Fat   22g

Protein   8 g

Sodium   14mg

Fiber   11g

Carbohydrates   15g

Sugar   1g

Weekend Western Omelet

PREPARATION: 10 MIN   **COOKING: 39 MIN**   **SERVING:**

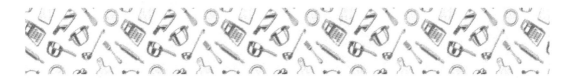

Ingredients:

8 large eggs

10 ounces smoked ham, finely chopped

4 tablespoons heavy whipping cream

1 small yellow onion, peeled and chopped

1 small green bell pepper, seeded and chopped

8 tablespoons unsalted butter, divided

1 cup shredded Cheddar cheese, divided

Directions:

In a large bowl, whisk eggs and mix in the ham and cream.

In a medium microwave-safe bowl, microwave the onion and pepper for 3 minutes.

In a medium skillet over medium-low heat, melt 2 tablespoons butter and quickly pour one-quarter of the egg mixture into skillet before it separates.

After 4–5 minutes, when entire bottom of egg mixture has cooked, add one-quarter of onion and pepper to center of omelet.

Use spatula to fold egg mixture in half onto itself. Let omelet finish cooking another 3–4 minutes.

Slide the fully cooked omelet onto a warmed plate. Top with one-quarter of shredded cheese.

Repeat process three more times for the remaining three omelets.

Nutrition:

Calories   593

Fat   46g

Protein   32g

Sodium   1,193mg

Fiber   1g

Carbohydrates   4g

Sugar   2g

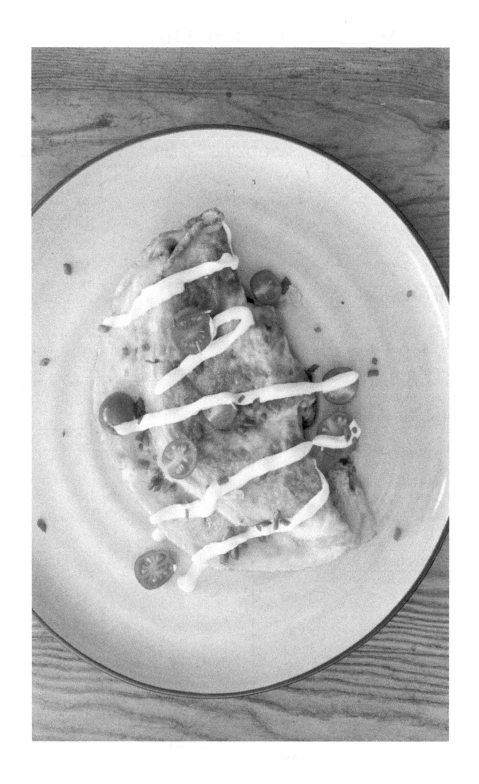

Christmas Soufflé

PREPARATION: 10 MIN   **COOKING: 35 MIN**   **SERVING:**

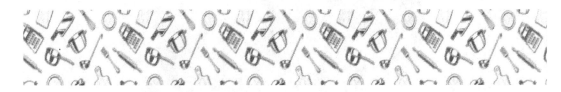

Ingredients:

½ tablespoon olive oil

1 medium onion, peeled and finely chopped

1½ teaspoons minced garlic

6 large eggs, whisked

6 ounces cured ham, finely cubed

1 cup shredded Cheddar cheese

½ cup heavy whipping cream

½ cup finely chopped tomato

½ cup finely chopped green onion

Directions:

Preheat oven to 400°F. Grease a 9" × 9" baking dish.

In a medium nonstick pan over medium heat, add oil, onion, and garlic. Cook 3–5 minutes while stirring until brown and soft. Remove from heat.

In a large mixing bowl, mix all ingredients. Pour into baking dish.

Bake 25–30 minutes until cooked all the way through.

Serve Christmas Soufflé while warm.

Nutrition:

1. Calories   287
2. Fat   21g
3. Protein   16g
4. Sodium   475mg
5. Fiber   1g
6. Carbohydrates   4g
7. Sugar   2g

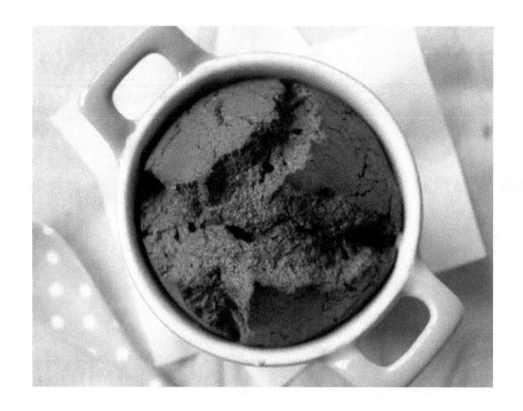

Counterfeit Bagels

PREPARATION: 15 MIN

COOKING: 17 MIN

SERVING:

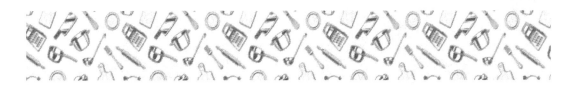

Ingredients:

1½ cups blanched almond flour

1 tablespoon baking powder

2½ cups shredded whole milk mozzarella cheese

2 ounces full-fat cream cheese, softened

2 large eggs, whisked

2 tablespoons Everything but the Bagel seasoning

1 tablespoon unsalted butter, melted

Directions:

Preheat oven to 400°F. Line a baking sheet with parchment paper.

In a small bowl, mix almond flour and baking powder.

In a medium microwave-safe bowl, mix mozzarella cheese, cream cheese, and whisked eggs.

Microwave cheese mixture 1 minute. Stir and microwave again 30 seconds. Let mixture cool until okay to handle.

Combine dry ingredients into cheese mixture. Work quickly, stirring with a sturdy spatula or bamboo spoon to create dough. Shape dough into approximately ¾"-thick snakes, and then form into ten bagels.

Place bagels on prepared baking sheet and sprinkle tops with seasoning. Bake 15 minutes until browning on top.

Remove bagels from oven, brush with melted butter, and serve.

Nutrition:

Calories   236

Fat   18g

Protein   11g

Sodium   548mg

Fiber   2g

Carbohydrates   5g

Sugar   1g

Starbucks Egg Bites

PREPARATION: 5 MIN

COOKING: 30 MIN

SERVING:

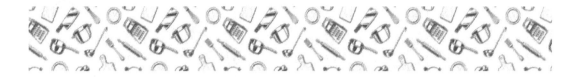

Ingredients:

5 large eggs, whisked

1 cup shredded Swiss cheese

1 cup full-fat cottage cheese

1/8 teaspoon salt

1/8 teaspoon black pepper

2 strips no-sugar-added bacon, cooked and crumbled

Directions:

Preheat oven to 350°F.

In a large bowl, whisk together eggs, Swiss cheese, cottage cheese, salt, and pepper.

Pour six equal amounts of mixture into well-greased muffin tins (or use cupcake liners).

Top with bacon bits.

Bake 30 minutes until eggs are completely cooked.

Remove Starbucks Egg Bites from oven and serve warm.

Nutrition:

Calories   182

Fat   11g

Protein   16g

Sodium 321mg

Fiber 0g

Carbohydrates 3g

Sugar 1g

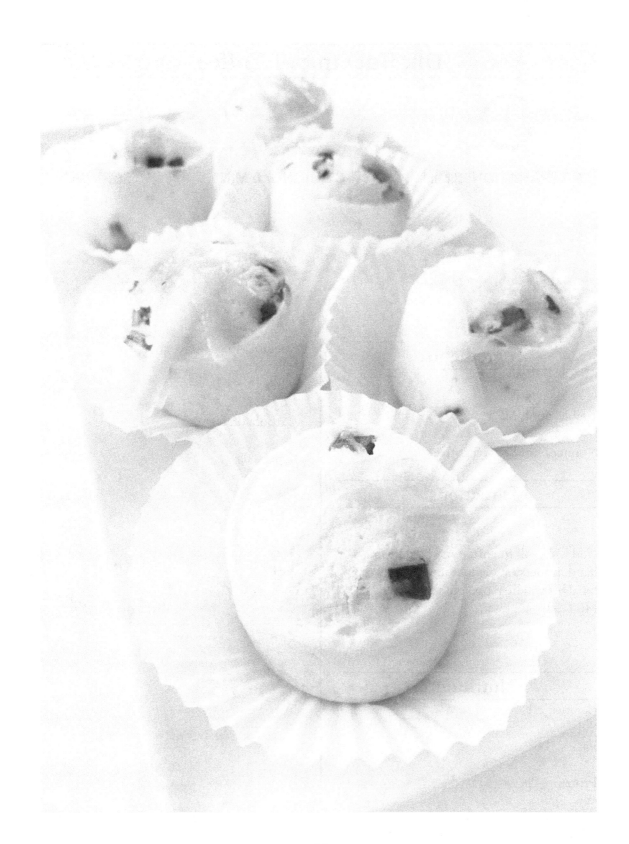

Dlk Bulletproof Coffee

PREPARATION: 2 MIN

COOKING: 0 MIN

SERVING:

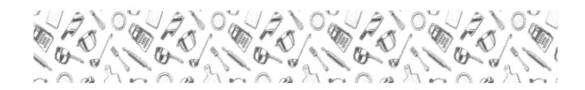

Ingredients:

1 tablespoon MCT oil

8 ounces hot brewed coffee

Directions:

Add MCT oil to coffee and blend using a hand immersion blender until froth whips up. This will help prevent the dreaded MCT oil "lip gloss."

Serve.

Nutrition:

Calories   132

Fat   14g

Protein   0g

Sodium 4mg

Fiber   0g

Carbohydrates 0g

Sugar   0g

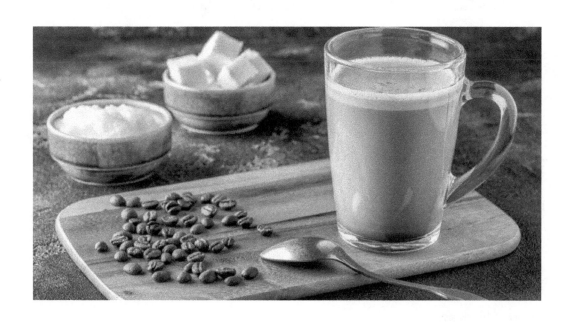

Radish Hash Browns

PREPARATION: 10 MIN   **COOKING: 40 MIN**   **SERVING:**

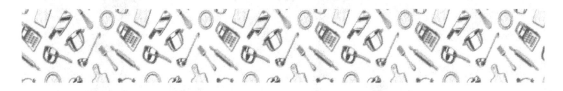

Ingredients:

2 pounds radishes, trimmed

4 tablespoons olive oil

1 large egg, whisked

1/8 teaspoon salt

1/8 teaspoon black pepper

Directions:

Shred radishes using a food processor or hand grater and squeeze out extra moisture using cheesecloth or clean dish towel.

In a medium skillet over medium heat, heat oil. Add radishes and stir often. Sauté 20–30 minutes until golden. Remove from heat and place into a medium bowl.

Stir whisked egg into bowl with salt and pepper.

Form ten small pancakes. Add back to hot skillet. Heat 3–5 minutes on each side until solid and brown.

Serve warm.

Nutrition:

Calories   63

Fat   6g

Protein   1g

Sodium   58mg

Fiber   1g

Carbohydrates   2g

Sugar   1g

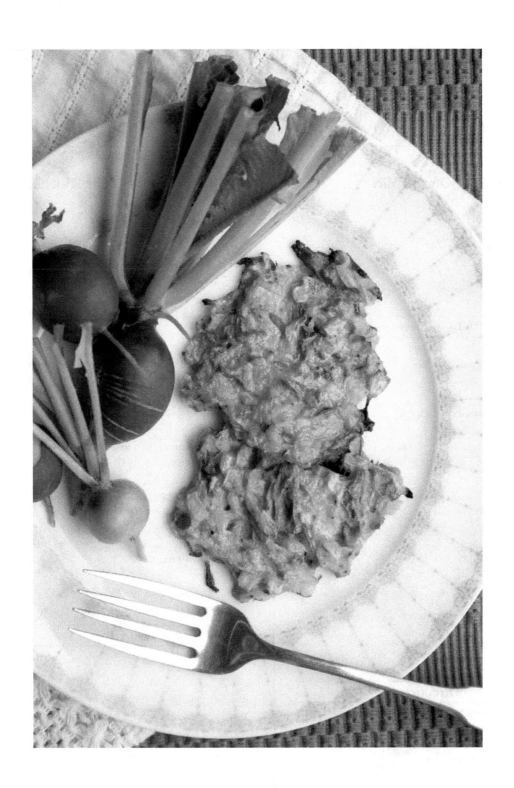

Easy Bake Keto Bread

PREPARATION: 10 MIN   **COOKING: 30 MIN**   **SERVING: 16**

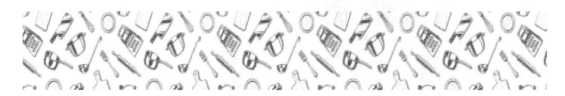

Ingredients:

7 whole eggs

4.5 oz. melted butter

2 Tbsp. warm water

2 tsp dry yeast

1 tsp. inulin

1 pinch of salt

1 tsp. xanthan gum

1 tsp. baking powder

1 Tbsp. psyllium husk powder

2 cups almond flour

Directions:

Preheat the oven to 340F.

In a bowl, mix almond flour, salt, psyllium, baking powder, and xanthan gum.

Make a well in the center of the mixture.

Add the yeast and inulin into the center with the warm water.

Stir the inulin and yeast with the warm water in the center and let the yeast activate, about 10 minutes.

Add in the eggs and melted butter and stir well.

Pour the mixture into a loaf pan lined with parchment paper.

Allow batter to proof in a warm spot covered for 20 minutes with a tea towel.

Place in the oven and bake until golden brown, about 30 to 40 minutes.

Cool, slice, and serve.

Nutrition:

Calories: 140

Fat: 13g

Carb: 3g

Protein: 3g

Keto Cloud Bread Cheese

PREPARATION: 5 MIN

COOKING: 30 MIN

SERVING: 12

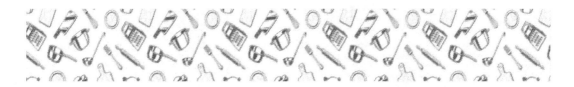

Ingredients

for cream cheese filling:

1 egg yolk

½ tsp. vanilla stevia drops for filling

8 oz. softened cream cheese

Base egg dough:

½ tsp. cream of tartar

1 Tbsp. coconut flour

¼ cup unflavored whey protein

3 oz. softened cream cheese

¼ tsp. vanilla stevia drops for dough

4 eggs, separated

Directions:

Preheat the oven to 325F.

Line two baking sheets with parchment paper.

In a bowl, stir the 8 ounces cream cheese, stevia, and egg yolk.

Transfer to the pastry bag.

In another bowl, separate egg yolks from whites.

Add 3 oz. cream cheese, yolks, stevia, whey protein, and coconut flour. Mix until smooth.

Whip cream of tartar with the egg whites until stiff peaks form.

Fold in the yolk/cream cheese mixture into the beaten whites.

Spoon batter onto each baking sheet, 6 mounds on each. Press each mound to flatten a bit.

Add cream cheese filling in the middle of each batter.

Bake for 30 minutes at 325F.

Nutrition:

1. Calories: 120
2. Fat: 10.7g
3. Carb: 1.1g
4. Protein: 5.4g

Keto Cloud Bread

PREPARATION: 10 MIN   **COOKING: 20 MIN**   **SERVING: 12**

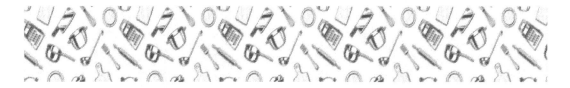

Ingredients:

3 tbsp. cream cheese

3 eggs

½ tsp. sea salt

¼ tsp. baking powder

¼ tsp. pepper

Directions:

Preheat oven to 350F.

Add egg yolks and cream cheese into a bowl and mix with a hand mixer.

In another bowl, add egg whites, pepper, salt and baking powder and mix for 5 minutes or until stiff peaks form.

Add the egg yolk mixture and egg white mixture together until mixed well.

Transfer mixture into a loaf pan and place into the prepared oven.

Bake for 15 to 20 minutes, or until lightly golden.

Nutrition:

Calories: 28

Fat: 2g

Carb:0 g

Protein: 2g

Cheesy Keto Sesame Bread

PREPARATION: 5 MIN   **COOKING: 30 MIN**   **SERVING: 8**

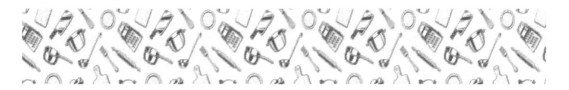

Ingredients:

1 tsp. sesame seeds

1 tsp. baking powder

1 tsp. salt

2 Tbsp. ground psyllium husk powder

1 cup almond flour

4 Tbsp. sesame or olive oil

7 ounces cream cheese

4 eggs

Sea salt

Directions:

Preheat the oven to 400F.

Beat the eggs until fluffy. Add cream cheese and oil until combined well.

Set the sesame seeds aside and add the remaining ingredients.

Grease a baking tray. Spread the dough in the greased baking tray. Allow it to stand for 5 minutes.

Baste dough with oil and top with a sprinkle of sesame seeds and a little sea salt.

Bake in the oven at 400F until the top is golden brown, about 30 minutes.

Nutrition:

1. Calories: 282
2. Fat: 26g
3. Carb: 2g
4. Protein: 7g

Keto Almond Bread

PREPARATION: 10 MIN　　**COOKING: 30 MIN**　　**SERVING: 20**

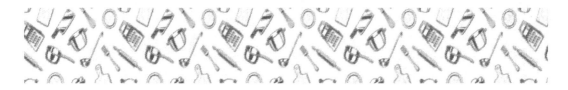

Ingredients:

1 ½ cups almond flour

3 tsp. baking powder

4 tbsp. butter, melted

¼ tsp. cream of tartar

6 eggs, whites and yolks separated

Pinch of salt

Directions:

Preheat the oven to 375F.

Grease a (8 x 4) inch loaf pan.

In a bowl, beat the cream of tartar and egg whites until soft peaks form.

Keep the mix on the side.

In a food processor, mix almond flour, salt, baking powder, egg yolks, and butter.

Add 1/3 cup egg whites to food processor and pulse until combined.

Add rest of the egg whites and mix until combined.

Pour into the prepared loaf pan and bake for 30 minutes.

Cool, slice, and serve.

Nutrition:

Calories: 271

Fat: 22g

Carb: 6g

Protein: 5g

Quick Low-Carb Bread Loaf

PREPARATION: 45 MIN　　**COOKING: 40 - 45 MIN**　　**SERVING: 16**

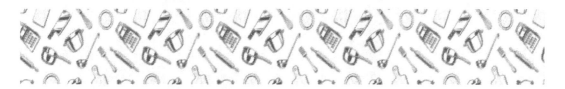

Ingredients:

2/3 cup coconut flour

½ cup butter, melted

3 Tbsp. coconut oil, melted

1 1/3 cup almond flour

½ tsp. xanthan gum

1 tsp. baking powder

6 large eggs

½ tsp. salt

Directions:

Preheat the oven to 350F. Cover the bread loaf pan with baking paper.

Beat the eggs until creamy.

Add in the coconut flour and almond flour, mixing them for 1 minute. Next, add the xanthan gum, coconut oil, baking powder, butter, and salt and mix them until the dough turns thick.

Put the completed dough into the prepared line of the bread loaf pan.

Place in oven and bake for 40 to 45 minutes. Check with a knife.

Slice and serve.

Nutrition:

Calories: 174

Fat: 15g

Carb: 5g

Protein: 5g

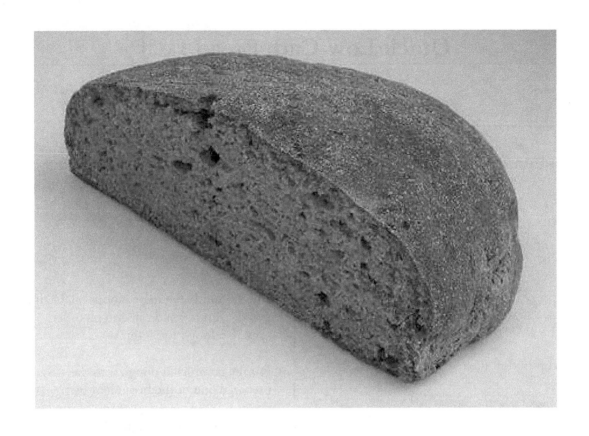